STAYING

HEALTHY

EAT WELL!

Miriam Moss

Wayland

STAYING HEALTHY

BE POSITIVE!
BODY CARE
EAT WELL!
KEEP FIT!

Series editor: Kathryn Smith
Series designer: Helen White

First published in 1992 by
Wayland (Publishers) Ltd
61 Western Road, Hove
East Sussex, BN3 1JD, England

British Library Cataloguing in Publication Data

Moss, Miriam
Eat Well. – (Staying Healthy Series)
I. Title II. Series
613.2

ISBN 0 7502 0369 2

Typeset by White Design.
Printed by Canale & C.S.p.A., in Turin.
Bound by A.G.M. in France.

CONTENTS

HEALTHY EATING

Why do we need food?

We need food to give us energy. When you haven't eaten for a while your stomach feels hot and empty and you start to feel listless. This is your body telling you that it needs more fuel to burn up so that you can remain active and energetic.

The food you eat is also used to make new body cells and to replace worn-out cells. The right kind of food also helps to fight infection and protect us from disease.

Do you eat well?

We are what we eat, and it follows that our eating habits must therefore affect our health. You can damage your health by eating badly. But if you eat the right kind of food in the correct quantities, then your body has more chance of staying healthy.

Which are your favourite foods? Eating habits come in all shapes and sizes. You may be a snacker who likes to pick and nibble but who rarely eats a large meal.

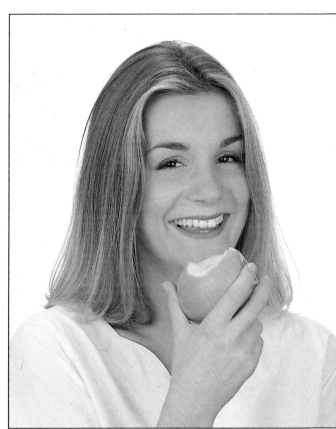

▶ Food is full of energy. It's fuel for life.

◀ If you feel hungry between meals try to snack on raw fruit and vegetables.

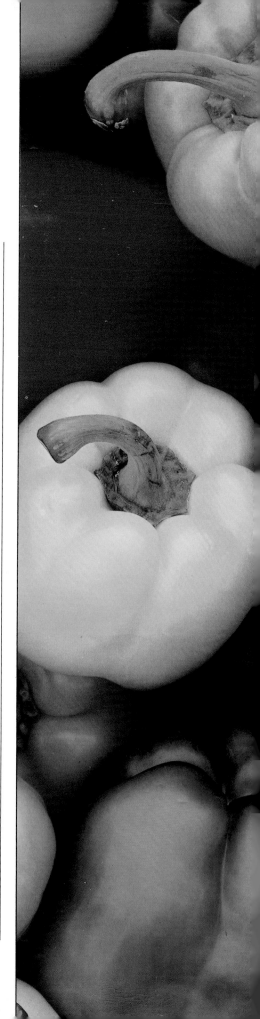

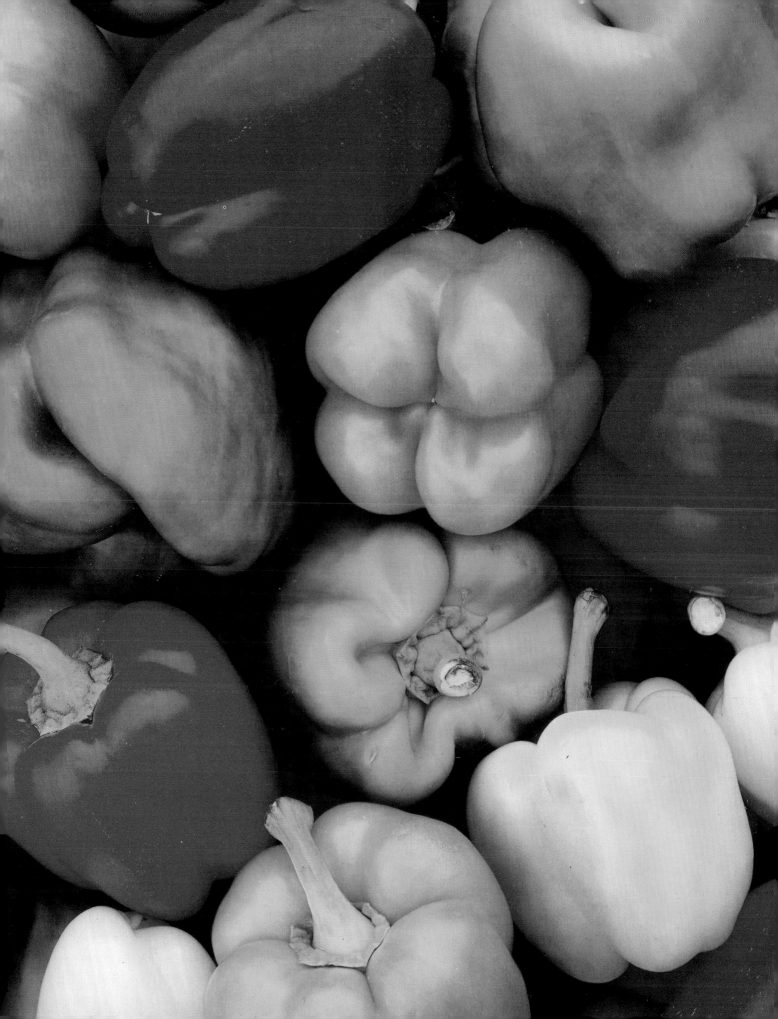

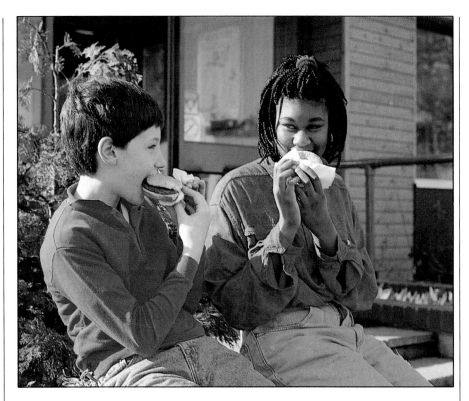

Perhaps you have a sweet tooth; you're someone who has to have just one more chocolate bar to satisfy that craving for sugar. Or you could be someone who eats out of boredom. This book discusses what you need to eat to remain healthy. It also talks about some of the dangers involved in eating the wrong kind of foods. The aim is to acquire good, healthy eating habits and to keep eating a well balanced diet for the rest of your life.

What is health?

Health is very difficult to define but we have to discover what we're aiming for. Looking at glossy magazines you might think that health is only about beauty and fitness. But someone can have a lean, muscular body and beautiful hair when their internal organs are in a very bad state.

▲ With today's busy lifestyle, it's very tempting to snack on fast food rather than make yourself a more nutritious meal.

▼ This picture shows how much land is needed to rear cattle for meat production. Compare it to the picture on p7.

Staying healthy is not just to do with eating healthily. It involves far more than this. Having good health involves eating well and exercising regularly to keep your body strong, supple and full of stamina. Health is the condition of both your body and your mind. Your health affects your social life too, because if you feel good about yourself then you also feel good about others.

Food for all?

There is enough food produced in the world to feed everybody, yet over half the people in the world do not have enough to eat. Some even die of starvation. It's a sad fact that health and wealth are strongly related. Poor people often go without food because they cannot afford to buy expensive food in short supply. Crops don't always grow where they are needed most.

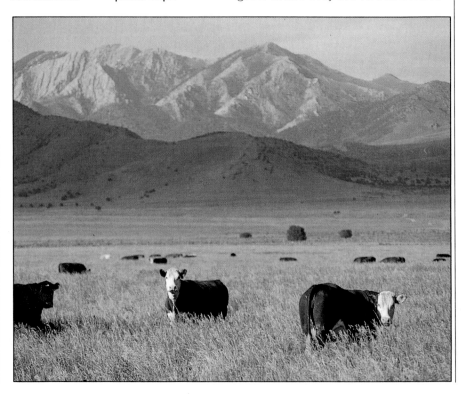

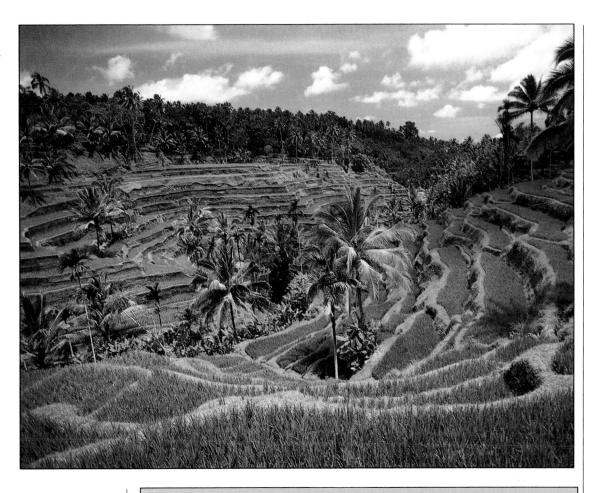

► These terraced rice fields in Indonesia show how effectively land can be used for farming. By terracing the slopes the farmers increase the area of land available to grow rice on.

Much of the world's food is grown in the USA, Europe and Australia. The United Nations have set a target date of the year 2000 for 'health for all' – basic health care for everyone. It's easy to think of health as other people's responsibility, but you can do your bit to help those less fortunate than yourself.

Developing countries often grow large cash crops for countries like Britain and the USA, such as coffee, instead of using land to grow food for themselves. People in richer, developed countries can change their eating habits, to lessen this demand for cash crops, so that vital resources can be left available for people who desperately need them.

Too much and too little

The amount of food you eat affects your health. Too little food leads to malnutrition. Too much food also leads to serious health problems. There is more obesity (a cause of heart disease) in rich countries now than ever before because of diets which are high in animal fats and sugar. Cutting down on animal fats, such as those in meat and dairy products, and eating more fresh, raw fruit and vegetables which retain vital vitamins and minerals, improves your diet. Most people in the world are vegetarian. Many people in developing countries enjoy a varied, healthy diet based on vegetables, fish and fruit. Others only have access to a diet lacking in essential vitamins and minerals. This leads to poor bone formation and related illnesses.

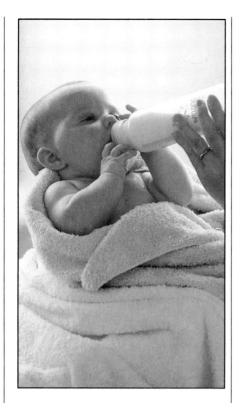

It's very important to eat the right amount and type of food as you grow up. When you were a baby you needed foods high in protein and carbohydrates for the intensive growth that you underwent in the first few months of your life. As an adolescent undergoing enormous body changes, you need to eat plenty of energy-giving food and proteins for growth. When you are much older you will need less food, but just like at other stages in your life, you'll need a diet which offers the full range of vitamins and minerals essential for health.

Food and illness

Just as what you eat can make you healthy, so what you eat can make you ill. Your warm, moist kitchen is a very good place for germs to multiply. This is why it is essential to follow the basic rules of hygiene, such as washing your hands before preparing and eating food. Bacteria and other germs are sometimes present in food. Salmonella is found in chickens, listeria in certain cheeses, brucellosis in meat and tuberculosis in milk. Better live-stock health and pasteurised milk do avoid these risks to health, but germs can grow easily inside food that is not stored at the right temperature. Contamination by these germs can result in food poisoning and stomach upsets. Cooking foods such as eggs and chicken thoroughly helps to kill these germs. In many parts of the world a lack of hygiene in processing water for domestic use leads to serious contamin-ation of water systems, which can cause disease and epidemics.

What happens to my food?

Your body needs the energy which is stored up in food to keep it running. But the body cannot use food just as it is to repair old cells and grow new ones. Your body needs to digest the food first, to break the large molecules in food down into smaller, simpler ones. Digestion starts in the mouth when you chew up food and mix it with your saliva. (Did you know that you can make up to 1.5 litres of saliva a day?) The enzymes, or chemicals in your saliva help to break down the food so that it can be digested.

The digestive juices in your stomach, the acids and enzymes released there, continue this pulping process. Your stomach can hold about a litre of food.

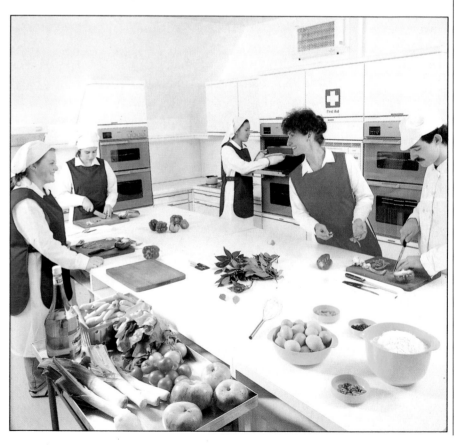

It remains there for about three hours before it is pushed into your small intestine, which is 6 -7 metres long. The food is now a thin liquid.

More enzymes are added with bile from the liver. The bile breaks down the fats into fatty acids and glycerol. Proteins are broken down into amino acids, whilst carbohydrates become sugars, such as glucose. These are all nutrients – the simple molecules that the body can use, and they pass through the intestine wall into your blood stream, where they are used to nourish your body.

The remaining food has the water taken out of it by the large intestine, which is about a metre long. The remaining waste material is passed out of the body. The whole digestive process takes between ten and twenty hours.

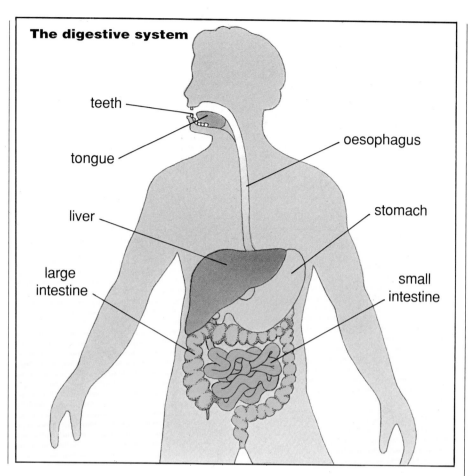

The digestive system

teeth

tongue

liver

large intestine

oesophagus

stomach

small intestine

▲ ABOVE
A diagram showing the major components of the digestive system.

◀ OPPOSITE TOP
When you were younger it was someone else's responsibility to make sure you had enough of the right kind of food to eat. Now it's up to you!

◀ OPPOSITE
Food in restaurants has to be prepared to strict standards of hygiene. How careful are you when you prepare food?

▶ Regular exercise helps your digestive system to work more efficiently.

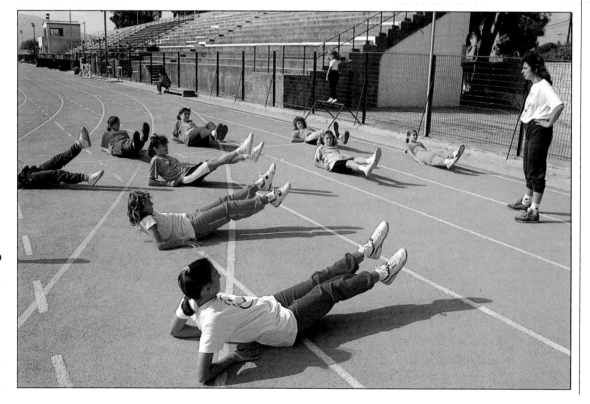

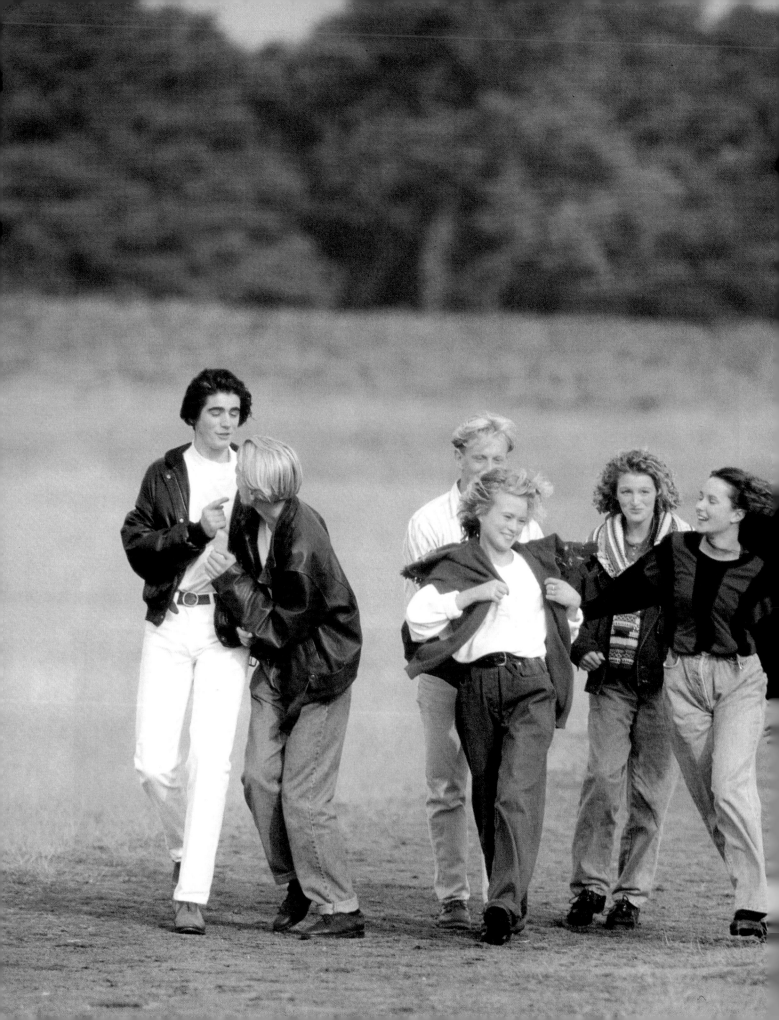

FEELING GOOD

It's your responsibility

Your health is your responsibility. It's all up to you. You choose whether to smoke and drink alcohol. You choose what you want to eat and how much you exercise.

Once you've decided to take responsibility for your diet you need to have a look at your daily intake. Make a note of what you consume over a few days and see how it shapes up. If you need to change to better eating habits it has to be done on a permanent basis. Watch out for food and drink advertisements! Don't be taken in or tempted by those that try to persuade you to eat food that is bad for you.

◀ You are what you eat ... and what you eat is your choice. A healthy diet is an essential part of feeling and looking good.

▶ Take responsibility for your own diet. When cooking for yourself and others think carefully about creating a nutritionally balanced meal.

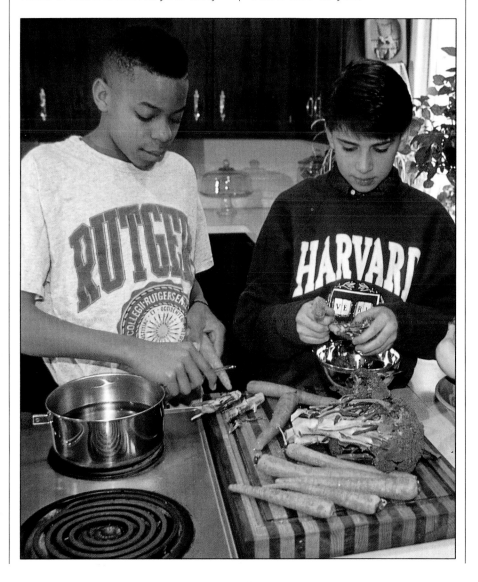

Exercise and health

Concentrating on one aspect of your health, such as your eating, is fine for a time but being really healthy means that you need to look after your body's fitness, and the health of your mind. Regular exercise is essential for real fitness. Exercise gives you a sense of well-being and helps you to relax. It also keeps your heart and lungs healthy as well as being a great way to meet people. Exercise burns off any excess calories that will otherwise be stored as fat by your body. So it helps you stay in good shape.

You can increase the amount of exercise you take very cheaply by just starting to walk or cycle instead of going by car or taking the bus. Check out your local sports centre or gym and join an exercise class. Whatever you choose to do, remember it has to be fun and it has to be regular. Two ways to ensure that you keep it up is to arrange to exercise with a friend and to make sure you choose something that you both enjoy. Try to exercise two or three times a week for about twenty minutes. Make sure that getting there doesn't require a long journey and that it isn't dependent on the weather. Don't stop there! Move on and try out some of the range of games and activities that are available.

Rest, relaxation and sleep

Being on the go all day and then burning the candle all night is not a recipe for health. A healthy person is one who recognizes the importance of rest, relaxation and sleep. If you have a late night, make up for lost sleep the next night. Being tired means that you cannot function well. Your body needs time to mend and replace the wear and tear of everyday life. As well as making sure you allow your body rest and plenty of sleep, you also need to know how to relax.

Many people are not good at recognizing signs of stress and dealing with it. You know that feeling of being wound-up and tense.

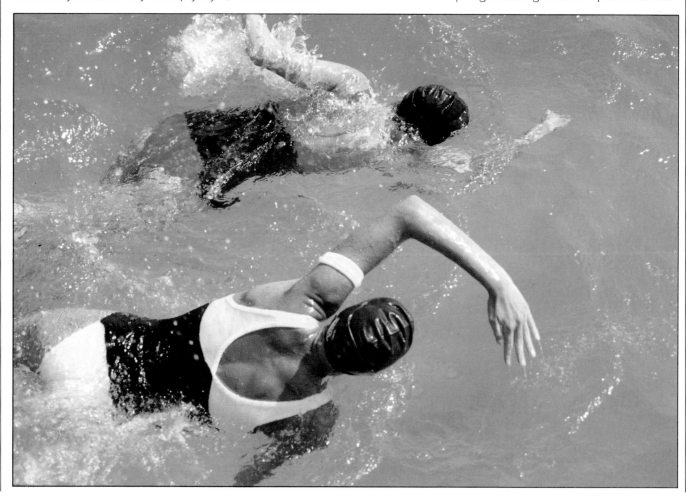

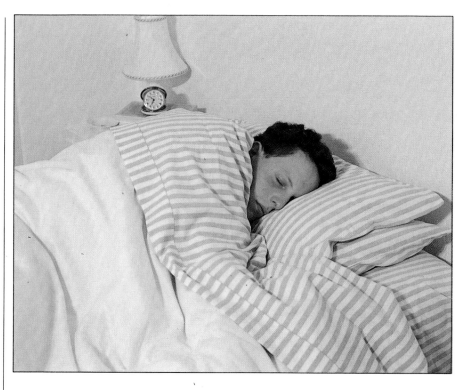

Your shoulders become tight and hunched. When this happens, opt out and give yourself some quiet time in which to unwind. Do something you enjoy, nurture yourself in a long, hot bath, then lie down, relaxing each muscle in your body in turn while you listen to some good music. Often talking about a problem which is giving you stress helps. Tell a friend what's bothering you. Whatever you do – don't ignore it! You'll find yourself pacing up and down later, unable to sleep. Feeling good about yourself is vital to feeling healthy, so don't forget to invest a little time each day learning to like yourself – it makes life much easier!

▲ ABOVE **On average most people need around eight hours sleep each night.**

◀ OPPOSITE **Swimming is one of the best forms of exercise for all round fitness.**

▶ **To calculate your stress level, add together the stress scores for those events which have happened to you in the past two months. Check your stress score result, to find out how stressed you are.**

Stress Score Results

0 – 6 A score of six or under suggests that you are not very stressed.

6 – 10 You are on the verge of being stressed and should look carefully at your lifestyle. Also consider anything which is worrying you particularly.

10 and over You are under considerably more stress than the average person. To avoid the risk of stress-related illness, you should consider carefully your techniques for dealing with stress.

Calculate your stress level

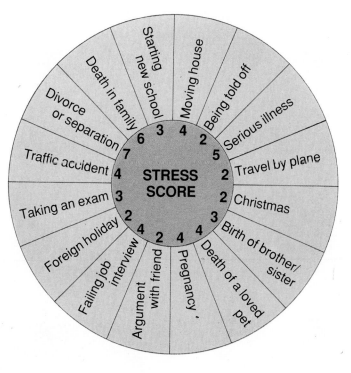

FITNESS FOOD

Balancing your diet
To stay alive we need oxygen, water, energy in the form of calories, vitamins and minerals and a small amount of carbohydrate. A mixed diet made up of reduced fat, sugar and salt and increased fibre will provide these essential nutrients. A balanced diet is one that contains the correct mix of nutrients to keep us in peak health.

To eat a varied, balanced diet you have to first eliminate bad habits. Start by avoiding snacks and junk food. Increase your fibre intake by eating more cereals, wholemeal bread, pasta and brown rice. Cut down on sugar, salt, fat and additives. Remember the key to a balanced diet is that too much of any one thing is not good for you, in other words – variety is the spice of life!

Try to increase the amount of fresh fruit, vegetables and pulses that you eat. Tinned and frozen food contain less vitamins and minerals. The way you prepare your food also makes a difference. Steamed food retains the flavour and goodness. Try to grill, steam or bake food and pour off excess fat while cooking meat rather than using it in sauces and gravies.

Your body is about two-thirds water so you need to drink plenty of water to remain healthy. This means about a litre a day which will help to flush out toxins and keep the system in good order.

▶ Different foods contain different nutrients. You need plenty of variety in your diet to remain healthy.

▼ Fresh fruit has a high water content and is rich in vitamins.

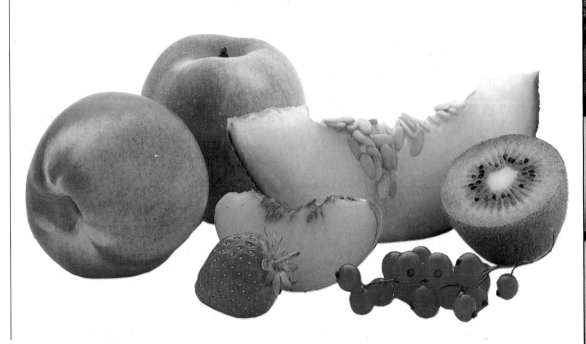

14

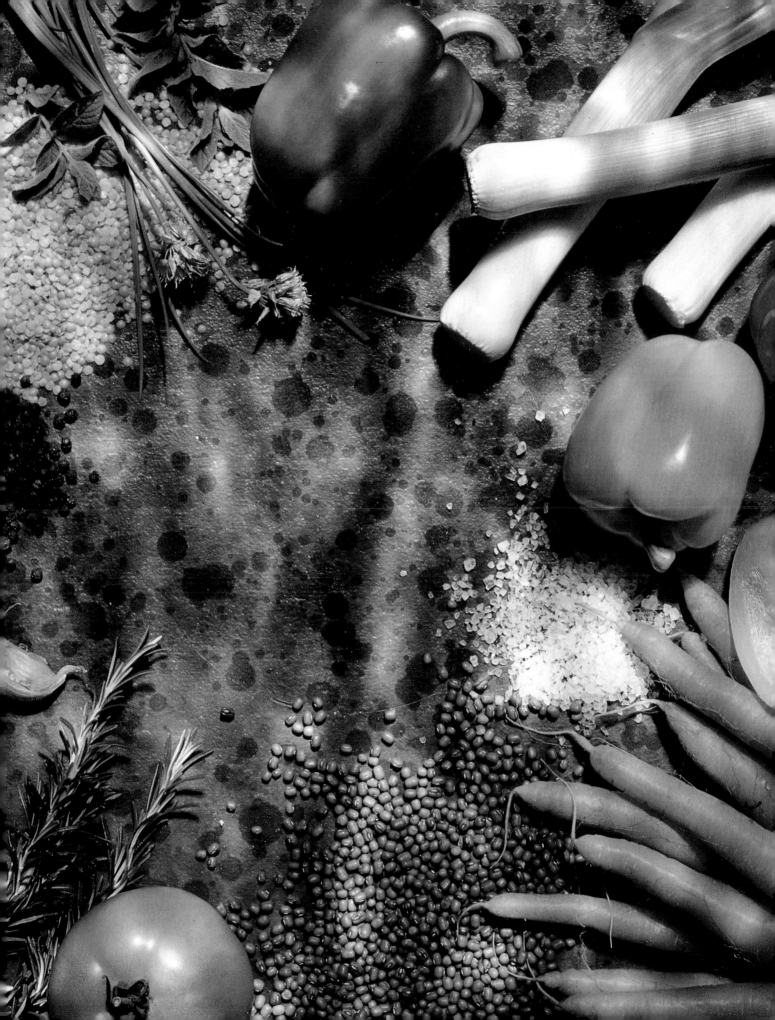

Enough is as good as a feast!
(The twice-a-week rule)

Here is a simple memory aid to help you eat a well-balanced diet that suits your digestive system and satisfies your nutritional needs.

Eat foods from each group no more than twice a week:

Group 1 meat and poultry
          2 fish
          3 eggs
          4 cheese
          5 food high in sugar (sweets and cakes)

Keep milk to about ½ litre a day and make up the rest of your diet from wholemeal bread, flour, cereals and grains, nuts and plenty of fresh fruit and vegetables.

Fight for fibre

Fibre is the indigestible matter in your diet. Lots of fibre in your diet increases the speed at which food passes through your intestines. Fibre helps to keep your bowels functioning healthily and protects you against bowel diseases. It also helps to fill you up. Good sources of fibre are bran, apricots and prunes, wholemeal bread, peas, beans and lentils and the skins of vegetables such as potatoes.

▼ Seafood is packed with protein. Many kinds of fish are low in saturated fat and high in oils which contain essential vitamins.

Check out carbohydrates

Most of your energy comes from carbohydrates. There are two main types: simple carbohydrates or sugars, and complex carbohydrates or starches. Experts now advise us to eat more of the complex carbohydrates found in foods such as potatoes, split peas and lentils, bread, pasta, rice, cereals, fruit and hard, leafy vegetables.

Protein packed

All your body's chemical reactions are dependent on proteins and all the body cells are made up of protein. It is found in foods such as lean meat, fish, dairy products, nuts, lentils, chick peas and beans. Protein supplies energy and helps your body build new cells and repair damaged body tissue.

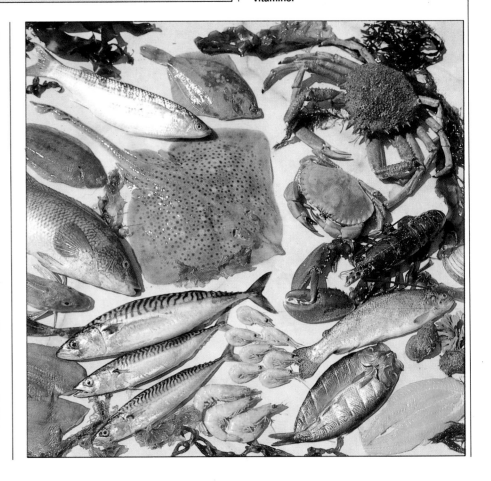

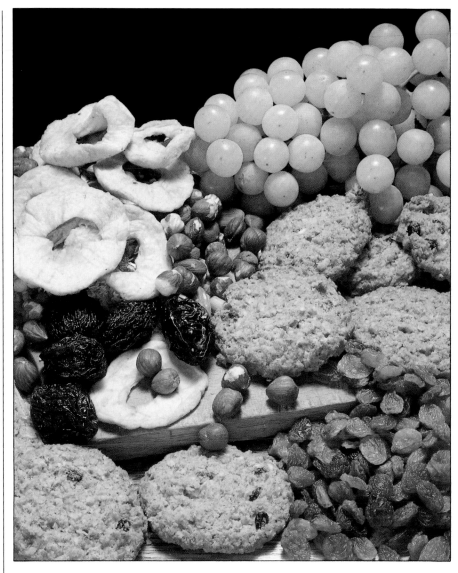

Vitamin and mineral vitality

Vitamins and minerals are very important substances needed by the body for various chemical reactions. The body cannot make most of them itself and so we have to get them from our food. However, they are only needed in very small amounts. The correct amounts are found in a balanced diet. Large amounts of, for example, vitamins A, D and B6 can damage your health so there is no point in overdoing your intake.

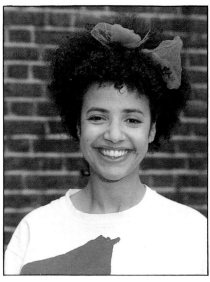

On the other hand, deficiencies in some important vitamins and minerals can lead to problems; for example iron deficiency leads to anaemia.

Vitamin A keeps your skin, teeth, hair and eyes healthy. It is also sometimes used to treat acne. You can find it in butter, eggs, cheese, spinach and broccoli. Vitamin C, found in citrus fruits, cabbage and sprouts, helps your body to fight infection. Try to eat some food containing vitamin C every day, as your body cannot store it. Foods rich in vitamin E are wholemeal products, green vegetables and brown rice. Vitamin D is found in oily kinds of fish and dairy products. It is also made by your body, using the action of sunlight on the oils of your skin. People who, for whatever reason, do not or cannot go out in the sunshine need to take special care that they get enough vitamin D from their food.

The most important minerals when you're growing fast, and for growth generally, are calcium and iron. Calcium is needed for the healthy development of teeth and bones, whilst iron is needed for healthy blood. Iron is found in eggs, liver, watercress, nuts and beans, and calcium is present in dairy products and green vegetables.

◄ **What you eat affects the way you look. Vitamin A, found in carrots, green leafy vegetables and dairy products, keeps your skin, teeth, hair and eyes healthy.**

▲ ABOVE LEFT **Fibre is essential for a healthy digestive system. All of these foods are high in fibre and make a good, healthy choice of snack between meals.**

CAREFUL EATING

Facts on fat

Too much fat is bad for you. By cutting down on your fat intake you can reduce your chances of developing heart disease and cancer, two of the biggest killers in most developed countries. There are three main types of fat: saturated, monounsaturated and polyunsaturated. Apart from coconut and palm oil, saturated fats are found in animal products such as milk, butter, cheese and meats. (The more saturated the fat the more solid it is.)

Saturated fats raise the cholesterol level in the blood which can lead to heart disease. Monounsaturated fats are found in nuts and fruit. Polyunsaturated fats are found in mackerel and pilchards. The oils used in salad dressings and for frying are also fats. If you want to reduce the fat in your diet try grilling rather than frying, and use skimmed milk, margarine high in polyunsaturates and low-fat yoghurt instead of cream. You can also use yoghurt to dress salads instead of oils.

Red meat has a high fat content so try cutting down on the amount you eat by eating more fish. Oily fish, such as mackerel, herring and trout, contain an acid which is believed to prevent coronary thrombosis. Some cheeses have a high fat content. Make sure the cheeses you eat are low-fat such as cottage or curd cheese. The rule 'too much of one thing isn't good for you' applies to eggs as well, so don't eat more than four eggs a week, including those used in cooking.

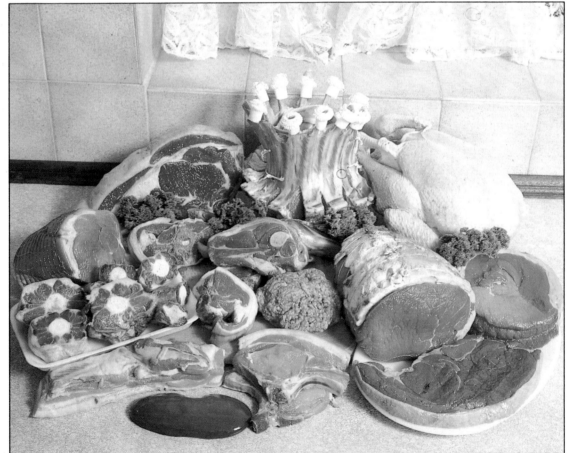

◀ Try to eat meat which is lean. The fat content of processed meat is difficult to detect just by looking. Check the food label to see how much fat a product contains.

▶ Many packaged foods like this mousse have been processed so much that they lose a lot of their original goodness. Additives are used to give them artificial colour, flavour and texture.

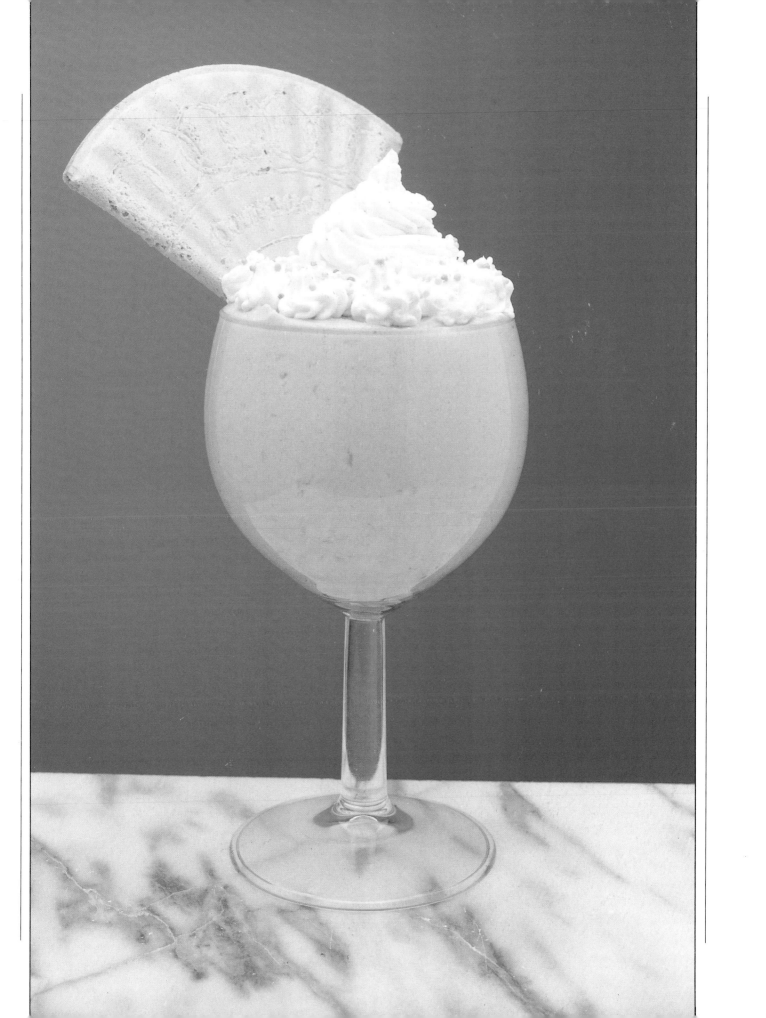

Action on additives

There may be links between what we eat and cancers. It is thought that the chemicals used in food can act as carcinogens (cancer-causing substances). The advice being given suggests that cutting down on the number of chemicals added to our food will mean that we are less likely to expose our bodies to these carcinogens. One way we can cut down on these chemicals is to remove pesticides on fruit and vegetables by washing them.

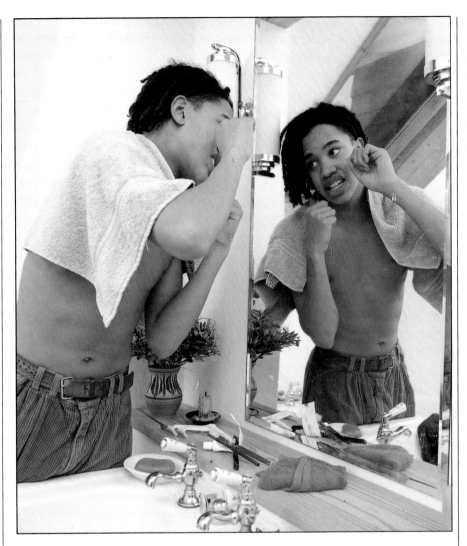

◄ It is important to take good care of your teeth, if you want to keep them all your life. Careful flossing every other day, together with daily brushing, helps to remove the build up of plaque on your teeth which causes tooth decay.

▼ You may be surprised at the number of additives used in factory processed foods such as biscuits and cakes. If you bake your own biscuits and cakes you can be sure of the ingredients used in them.

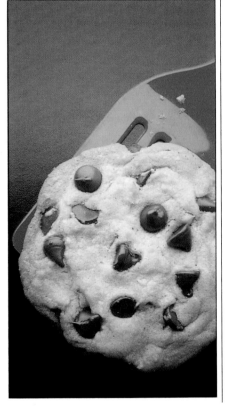

Hidden sugar and salt

Sugar provides energy, but it also causes our teeth to rot and contributes to high blood pressure, amongst other things. For this reason, it is good to be able to spot when we are eating sugar. Watch out for hidden amounts of sugar in cereals, fizzy drinks, mayonnaise, yoghurts and baked beans by checking the food labels. The ingredients used in the greatest quantities come first on the list. Labels may call sugar dextrose, fructose, sucrose, maltose, glucose or lactose – but it's all sugar! Try replacing sugary snacks with fruit or raw vegetables and use savoury spreads on bread.

Salt may make some people more likely to develop high blood pressure. You need to look carefully at packaged food to find the levels of salt in it (you will find this information on the ingredient label). You'll be surprised at how much is used for flavouring. When you cook try flavouring food with herbs instead of salt and avoid processed foods that contain large amounts of salt such as gravy, sauce mixes and even cereals, such as cornflakes.

Naturally fresh

Many people are concerned about the use of drugs such as antibiotics and hormones to speed up growth rates of livestock. These drugs are injected into animals, and in this way enter the food chain. Many also feel uneasy about irradiated food, where low doses of radiation are used to sterilize and preserve food in sealed packs. The long-term effects of radiation are not known. As a result more and more organic food is now on sale in shops and supermarkets, and a greater awareness has developed amongst the public about what they consume.

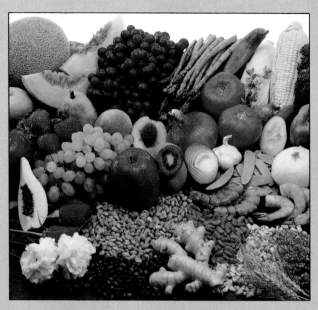

Also, we can eat fewer smoked meats which are high in nitrates, keep cling film away from fatty foods such as butter (which can be contaminated by the PVC) and avoid additives.

Additives have to be listed on ingredient labels of packaged food. They are used to brighten the colour of food, to flavour, sweeten, acidify, preserve or thicken it. (There are 1200 legal additives for ice-cream alone!) Many additives are harmless but some, for example tartrazine (an orange colouring) and sodium nitrate (a preservative) can cause allergic responses such as sickness, faintness and skin rashes in some people.

Cutting down

Coffee and tea contain the drug caffeine which is a stimulant. It perks you up but then leaves you more tired than before.

▼ Caffeine, found in tea and coffee, is a stimulant. If you want a drink before you go to bed at night, why not make a hot, milky drink which contains no caffeine.

▲ Although this selection of fruit and vegetables looks fresh and appetizing, you cannot tell which chemicals have been used to grow and preserve them.

Organically grown vegetables and fruit are never as brightly coloured or large as those grown using chemicals, but they have a much better flavour.

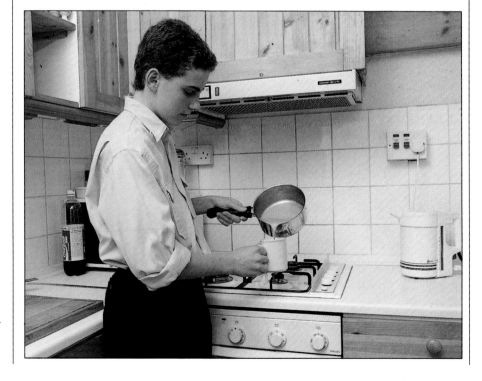

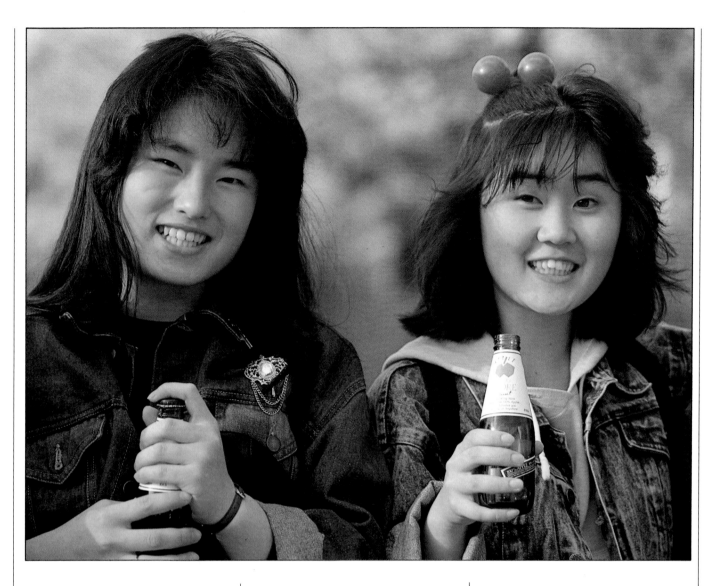

Too much caffeine can make you jumpy and tense and stop you sleeping well at night. You can buy decaffeinated coffee and tea, although some people question whether the chemicals used in decaffeination are as harmful as the caffeine itself. A growing number of people are enjoying a wide range of herbal teas which contain no caffeine.

Drinking too much alcohol causes problems to almost every system in your body as well as helping to destroy your social and family life. Alcohol is high in calories, so overuse often causes weight problems. It is a mild poison which is pumped around your body until it is neutralized by your liver. When it reaches your brain it affects your actions, your judgement, senses and speech. A unit of alcohol is about half a pint of beer or a standard glass of wine. Medical experts, aiming to stem the flow of alcohol-connected illnesses, advise drinking water to quench thirst, not alcohol, and to alternate alcohol with soft drinks at parties. The standard units recommended per week are twenty-one for men and fourteen for women, with three days a week without any alcohol at all.

Fast food

It's not surprising that young people who are growing fast and using up a lot of energy during the day become hungry between meals. Snacks between meals are not necessarily a bad thing; it just depends on what your snack consists of. If it's some biscuits or a bar of chocolate, it's full of sugar and high in calories but low in nutritional value.

What's really in it?

A breakdown of what a standard sesame bun, hamburger and chips really contain.

	Calories	Protein	Fibre	Fat
Sesame seed bun	170	9.8g	2.9g	7.3g
Hamburger	252	13.6g	0g	9.9g
Relish	30	0g	0g	0g
Small portion chips	288	3.7g	0g	15.2g

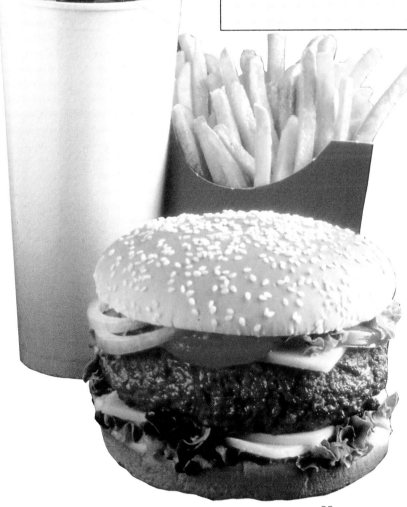

A lot of snacking means you could be heading towards being overweight and damaging your teeth. Snacking sensibly means eating brown bread sandwiches with sugarless fillings such as sugarless peanut butter, fruit, yoghurt, raw vegetables – raisins if you crave for something sweet.

Fast food chains provide constant snacks for millions of young people all over the world. The food for sale is often called 'junk' food. Some of it lives up to this name. It is highly processed, and contains little nutritional value. However, you can choose more nutritious, fibre-rich, low-fat fast food such as baked potatoes with low-fat fillings, salads or sandwiches made from wholemeal bread. Don't forget to choose fruit juice or sugar-free 'diet' drinks to go with your food.

EATING AND DIETS

Calories and energy

The energy that you need to function comes from the fat, carbohydrates and protein that you eat. A calorie is a measurement of energy. Fat contains the most calories per gram and protein the least. The number of calories you need just to keep your heart beating and your body at the right temperature depends on your age, size and sex, but the average is around 1500 calories. The number of calories needed after that depends on how active you are. The more exercise you take the more calories you need as you burn up the energy. Brainwork needs few calories. So if you are sitting around studying and eating a lot of calories, then you're going to put on weight!

The speed at which energy is used to keep your body working, to breathe and to pump the blood around, is called your basic metabolic rate, or BMR. Individual metabolic rates vary. Two people can eat the same amount of food and take the same amount of exercise and one may gain weight, whilst the other loses it.

Special diets

Dieting has become big business in the developed world and the variety of diets on offer is enormous. Crash dieting of any kind is not a sensible option. It just confuses your body's appetite control system.

Average daily calorie requirements

Children	1000-3000
Teenagers	2000-3000
Women (Sedentary)	2000
(active)	2300-4000
Men (Sedentary)	2500
(active)	3000-5000
Elderly people	1000-2000

▶ Dieting has become big business in the developed world. There is a huge variety of books and magazines on offer claiming to have the secret to weight loss.

▼ This waist stretching exercise stretches the muscles in the lower spine and keeps your waist trim. Stand with your legs apart and with your knees slightly bent. Move gently and slowly to the side, bending slightly forwards as you do so.

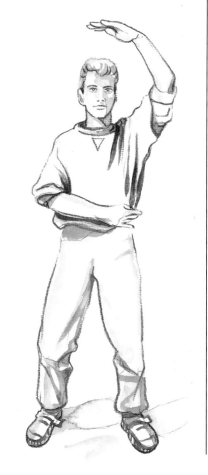
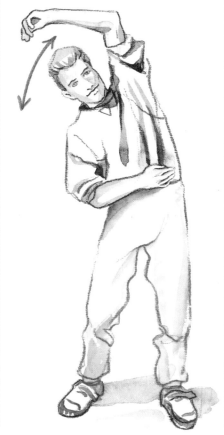

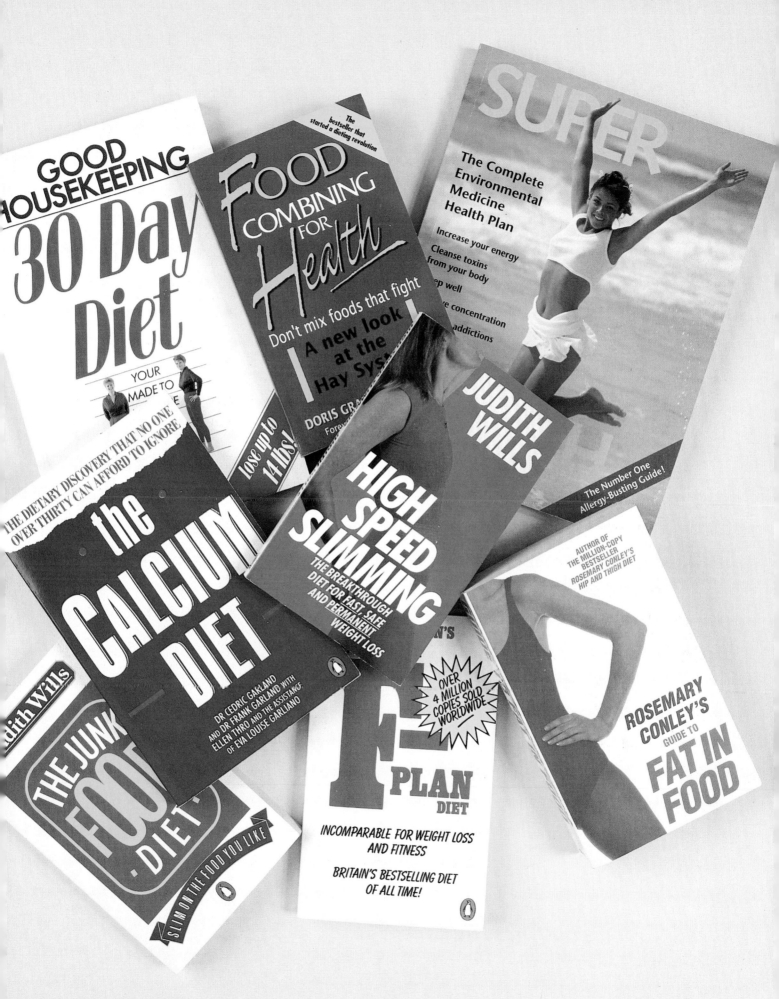

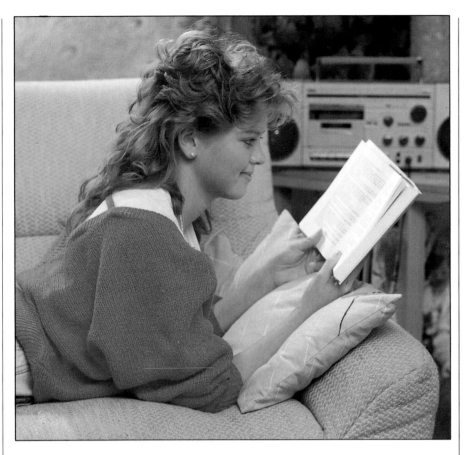

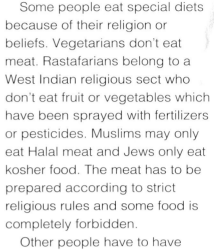

Some people eat special diets because of their religion or beliefs. Vegetarians don't eat meat. Rastafarians belong to a West Indian religious sect who don't eat fruit or vegetables which have been sprayed with fertilizers or pesticides. Muslims may only eat Halal meat and Jews only eat kosher food. The meat has to be prepared according to strict religious rules and some food is completely forbidden.

Other people have to have restricted diets for health reasons. Diabetics have the amount of sugar they eat carefully controlled. People suffering from asthma often have a special diet recommended to them.

Other people have allergic reactions. Those on gluten-free diets avoid gluten found in some cereals. Many people have allergic reactions to one kind of food, such as strawberries, shellfish or nuts, and have to avoid eating these.

Crash dieting causes water and stored sugar to be lost rather than fat. It also robs the body of vitamins and minerals. Trying out different diets without radically changing your eating habits for better, healthier ones is also a waste of time. You may lose weight but then as soon as you go back to your original habits the weight will slip back on.

If you really want to lose weight (and do you really need to?), then there is only one way: eat fewer calories and take more exercise. In practice more exercise and fewer calories per day is an easy regime to stick to, especially as exercise increases your metabolic rate. Obviously you need to stick to a good, balanced diet as well. Stay away from fats and don't bolt your food – take time over eating. Don't eat if you are not hungry – enough is as good as a feast!

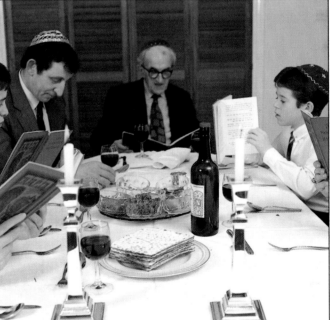

▲ TOP LEFT **Different activities burn up different amounts of calories. Less active pastimes such as reading, use up very few calories.**

◄ **What people eat is often dependent on religious or ethical beliefs. This family follows the Jewish religion, which states that the food they eat must be kosher.**

Eating disorders

Overeating and a lack of exercise are the most frequent causes of being overweight. Unused calories are stored as fat. Overweight people are more likely to get diabetes, high blood pressure and heart diseases than

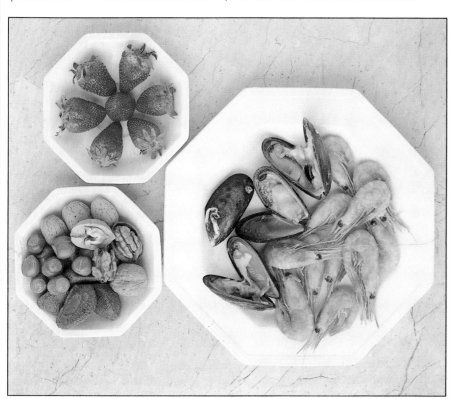

people of a normal weight because they put their hearts and joints under unnecessary strain. Eating for comfort or to compensate for some unsatisfied need is not uncommon. Unfortunately food and the need for comfort go together. Right from birth babies are fed to comfort them when they cry, so it is not surprising that food continues to be a comfort to some. People also eat too much out of boredom. Sometimes too much food and not enough exercise can be a sign of depression.

Anorexia nervosa

Weight gain and loss linked to eating disorders such as anorexia nervosa and bulimia nervosa may often be connected with unresolved emotional problems. There are about twenty times more female anorectics than males. Some experts believe anorexia hits the people who are more vulnerable to messages which tell them that they have to be perfect if they are to be loved and accepted by others. Anorectics have a very low opinion of themselves. They cannot let go and enjoy themselves but feel that at least they have power over their body weight by controlling it.

Anorexia can start as normal dieting which becomes compulsive. The less an anorectic eats, the less they want to eat. The more weight lost, the more terrified the anorectic becomes of gaining weight. The anorectic's body image is so distorted that they believe themselves to be fat even when they are dangerously underweight. They go to great lengths to avoid eating and, in extreme cases, need medical help and counselling to treat the disease and the underlining causes of it. The symptoms of anorexia nervosa can be: loss of periods in girls, loss of head hair and dry, rough skin.

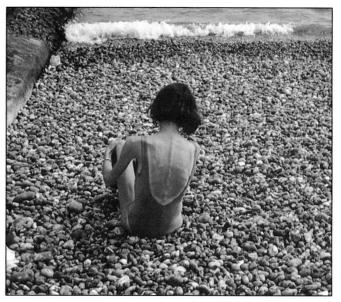

▲ TOP LEFT
A selection of foods which people are commonly allergic to. Food allergy sufferers experience a wide range of symptoms, including stomach cramps, feeling sick or rashes.

◄ Anorexia nervosa is an illness connected with emotional problems. An anorectic believes he or she still needs to lose weight, even when dangerously thin.

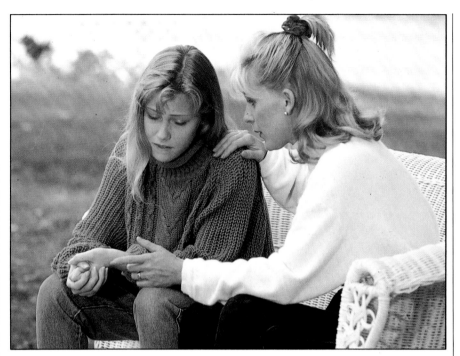

Their bingeing can involve enormous amounts of food. They punish themselves by purging their bodies of the food, and in extreme cases become exhausted or fall into a coma.

If you think someone you care about is suffering from one or other of these diseases, talk to someone you can trust about it and get help from the list of agencies at the back of this book. There are also many self-help groups where people with eating disorders can meet and talk about their problems.

Right for you

Many people worry about their weight, shape and size, constantly comparing themselves unfavourably with others. Some choose to go through life being discontented with the shape and appearance that they have been given, others accept themselves for what they are. There's no doubt that pressures from the

Bulimia nervosa

People suffering from bulimia eat huge quantities of usually sweet food, and then feel extremely ashamed, guilty and disgusted with themselves. Then they get rid of the food by being sick or taking laxatives. Bulimics give the impression of being happy and confident. Sufferers appear normal and often have an average weight. But they're over concerned by their weight and their shape. They can eat a lot without getting fat but their eating is quite out of control.

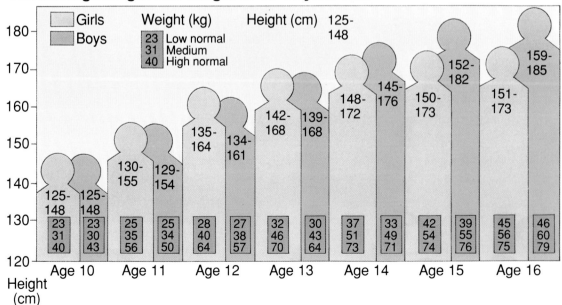

The average height and weight of 10-16 year olds

▲ TOP LEFT **If you are worried about something or someone, talk to a person you can trust.**

▶ OPPOSITE PAGE **The media continually presents us with images we cannot live up to. What do you think we can do about this?**

◀ **This chart shows the average height and weight of 10 – 16 year olds.**

media, fashion and culture are immense. We are constantly bombarded with body images which, to the average person in the street are impossible to achieve. How many people do you know with the figure and looks of a fashion model? Fashion dictates the perfect figure to us and then every few years changes its mind. One minute fashionable females must power dress, looking hard and androgynous. Next they're expected to look soft, full-figured and feminine, then athletic, muscle-toned and glowingly fit and healthy!

Males, on the other hand, have to quick change from a sensitive, romantic, artistic look to suddenly acquiring a body like a body builder.

The perfect figure is the one you have because real people come in all shapes and sizes! The right weight for you depends on what you are happiest with, as well as your height and build. (See the chart on p.28.) The aim is to eat well, enjoy your exercise and be happy with who you are!

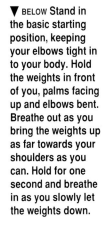

▼ BELOW **Stand in the basic starting position, keeping your elbows tight in to your body. Hold the weights in front of you, palms facing up and elbows bent. Breathe out as you bring the weights up as far towards your shoulders as you can. Hold for one second and breathe in as you slowly let the weights down.**

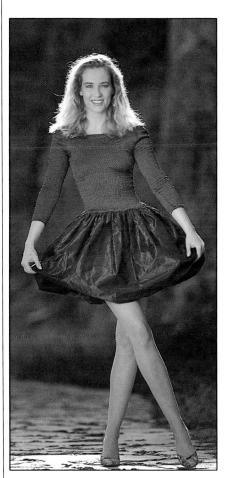

▶ **Regular exercise can help to tone up your body and keep it trim. These simple bicep curl exercises** will help to strengthen the biceps muscles in your arms and keep them well toned.

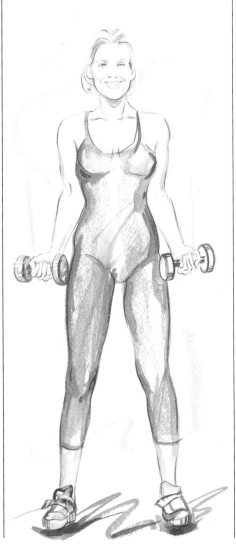

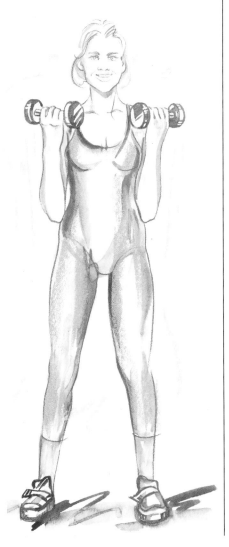

GLOSSARY

Additive Any substance added to food, such as colouring or flavouring.

Amino acid A group of compounds that contain the main molecules of proteins.

Androgynous Appearing to be both male and female.

Bacteria Organisms, many of which cause disease.

Calories Units of measurement of the energy in food.

Carbohydrate A substance found in food which gives energy.

Cholesterol A substance found in the body which, if there is too much, can block the arteries and cause a heart attack.

Deficiencies A lack, insufficiency or shortage of something.

Enzyme A substance produced by digestive glands which helps break down food during digestion.

Food chain The sequence where an organism feeds on another and is in turn eaten itself.

Glycerol A colourless, odourless, syrupy liquid.

Halal meat Meat killed according to Muslim law.

Kosher food Food prepared according to Jewish dietary laws.

Laxative A medicine which causes you to empty your bowels.

Malnutrition A lack of the right nutrition.

Neutralize To make something neutral.

Nitrate A substance containing nitric acid.

Obesity Excessively fat.

Organic Food grown without the use of pesticides or fertilizers.

Pesticide A chemical used for killing pests.

Protein A substance in food necessary for growth.

Pulses The edible seed of several green-leaved plants such as peas, beans and lentils.

Saliva A clear fluid produced by glands in the mouth to help with digestion.

Toxin A poisonous substance.

United Nations An international organization of independent states.

BOOKS TO READ

You and Your Fitness and Health by Kate Fraser and Judy Tatchell
(Usborne, 1986)
Exercise and Fitness by Brian R Ward (Franklin Watts, 1988)
Everygirl's Lifeguide by Miriam Stoppard (Dorling Kindersley, 1987)
Health and Fitness in Focus by Hilary Tunnicliffe (Franklin Watts, 1991)
Choosing Health by Alan Collinson (Cloverleaf, an imprint of Evans
Brothers Limited, 1991)
People and Energy by Jan Burgess (Macmillan Ltd, 1987)
Diet and Health by Ida Weekes (Wayland, 1991)
Health and Food by Dorothy Baldwin (Wayland, 1987)
Food and Hygiene by Pete Sanders (Franklin Watts, 1990)

FURTHER INFORMATION

Look After Yourself Project Centre
Christ Church College
Canterbury, Kent CT1 1QU
Tel: (0227) 455564
They will tell you the number of
your regional office.

Health Education Authority
78 New Oxford Street
London, WC1A 1AH

British Heart Foundation
14 Fitzhardinge Street
London, W1H 4DH

For help and advice on giving up
smoking, contact:
Action on Smoking and Health
(ASH)
5-11 Mortimer Street
London, W1N 7RH

A A A (Action Against Allergy)
43 The Downs
London, SW20 8HG

Anorexic Aid (Support and
information for anorectics and
their families)
The Priory Centre
11 Priory Road
High Wycombe
Bucks., HP13 6SL

Alcoholics Anonymous
PO Box 514
11 Redcliffe Gardens
London, SW10 9BQ

Fresh Fruit and Vegetable
Information Bureau
126-128 Cromwell Road
London, SW7 4ET

Food Commission
88 Old Street
London, EC1

INDEX

Picture Acknowledgements

J. Allan Cash 17 (top); Cephas 4 (left, Mick Rock), 6 (bottom, Mick Rock), 22; Chapel Studios 10, 21, 25; Eye Ubiquitous 9 (Julia Waterlow), 13; Jeff Greenberg 11; S&R Greenhill 27 (top); Tony Stone Worldwide 4/5 (L. Lefkowitz), 7 (D. Austen), 12 (C. Harvey), 14 (I. O'Leary), 15 (T. Wood), 21 (J. Camban); Topham 17 (bottom); Wayland Picture Library 6 (top), 16,18, 19, 20 (top), 27; Zefa 8 (top, bottom), 20 (bottom), 23, 26 (top, bottom), 28 (top, bottom). Artwork on pages 24 and 29 by Debbie Hinks. Artwork on pages 9, 13 and 28 by Marilyn Clay.